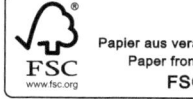

Dr. Inam Danish Khan

Rapid Diagnosis of Dengue Outbreaks in Resource Limited Facilities

Anchor Academic
Publishing

Khan, Inam Danish: **Rapid Diagnosis of Dengue Outbreaks in Resource Limited Facilities**, Hamburg, Anchor Academic Publishing 2017

Buch-ISBN: 978-3-96067-100-8
PDF-eBook-ISBN: 978-3-96067-600-3
Druck/Herstellung: Anchor Academic Publishing, Hamburg, 2017

Bibliografische Information der Deutschen Nationalbibliothek:
Die Deutsche Nationalbibliothek verzeichnet diese Publikation in der Deutschen Nationalbibliografie; detaillierte bibliografische Daten sind im Internet über http://dnb.d-nb.de abrufbar.

Bibliographical Information of the German National Library:
The German National Library lists this publication in the German National Bibliography. Detailed bibliographic data can be found at: http://dnb.d-nb.de

All rights reserved. This publication may not be reproduced, stored in a retrieval system or transmitted, in any form or by any means, electronic, mechanical, photocopying, recording or otherwise, without the prior permission of the publishers.

Das Werk einschließlich aller seiner Teile ist urheberrechtlich geschützt. Jede Verwertung außerhalb der Grenzen des Urheberrechtsgesetzes ist ohne Zustimmung des Verlages unzulässig und strafbar. Dies gilt insbesondere für Vervielfältigungen, Übersetzungen, Mikroverfilmungen und die Einspeicherung und Bearbeitung in elektronischen Systemen.

Die Wiedergabe von Gebrauchsnamen, Handelsnamen, Warenbezeichnungen usw. in diesem Werk berechtigt auch ohne besondere Kennzeichnung nicht zu der Annahme, dass solche Namen im Sinne der Warenzeichen- und Markenschutz-Gesetzgebung als frei zu betrachten wären und daher von jedermann benutzt werden dürften.

Die Informationen in diesem Werk wurden mit Sorgfalt erarbeitet. Dennoch können Fehler nicht vollständig ausgeschlossen werden und die Diplomica Verlag GmbH, die Autoren oder Übersetzer übernehmen keine juristische Verantwortung oder irgendeine Haftung für evtl. verbliebene fehlerhafte Angaben und deren Folgen.

Alle Rechte vorbehalten

© Anchor Academic Publishing, Imprint der Diplomica Verlag GmbH
Hermannstal 119k, 22119 Hamburg
http://www.diplomica-verlag.de, Hamburg 2017
Printed in Germany

PREFACE

Dengue, a viral disease known since long, continues to occur in endemic and epidemic proportions affecting half of the world population living in tropical developing world. Year after year, epidemics cripple the developing nation health systems due to high morbidity and limited mortality. There is a felt need of rapid diagnostic techniques for resource limited countries, laboratories and communities to prevent serious complications. No anti-dengue vaccines or therapy exist for dengue.

This book is intended to present information on dengue in a concise and simple manner for it to be suitable to academia, researchers and fellows, infectious diseases specialists, clinical microbiologists, virologists, residents and students, laboratory managers and industry leaders, in tropical developing economies.

I stand grateful for the mentorship of my teachers, encouragement of my family, support of my colleagues and friends, and diligence of the editorial team at Diplomica Publishing Group towards this endeavour.

Major Dr Inam Danish Khan

TABLE OF CONTENTS

Preface 1

List of Abbreviations 4

Chapter 1: Introduction 7

Chapter 2: Etymology, History and Epidemiology of Dengue 8

Chapter 3: Virology of Dengue 12

Chapter 4: Dengue Vectors and Transmission 15

Chapter 5: Dengue viral infection and Host Factors 19

Chapter 6: Immunological Response to Dengue 20

Chapter 7: Clinical Presentation of Dengue 24

Chapter 8: Laboratory Diagnosis of Dengue 30

Chapter 9: Rapid Diagnosis in Epidemic Scenario 38

References 41

LIST OF ABBREVIATIONS

ADE	-	Antibody Dependent Enhancement
CFT	-	Complement Fixation Test
CTLA4	-	Cytotoxic T-Lymphocyte Antigen 4
CLEC5A	-	C-type lectin domain family 5 member A
cDNA	-	complimentary Deoxyribonucleic Acid
dNTP	-	Deoxyribonucleotide triphosphate
DC-SIGN	-	Dendritic Cell-Specific Intercellular adhesion molecule -3-Grabbing Non-integrin
DFA	-	Direct Fluorescent Antibody
DEPC	-	Diethylpyrocarbonate
FcγR	-	Fcγ receptor
G6PD	-	Glucose 6 Phosphate Dehydrogenase
GRP78	-	Member of the HSP family of molecular chaperones
HI	-	Haemagglutination Inhibition
HSP	-	Heat Shock Proteins
IFN	-	Interferon
NASBA	-	Nucleic Acid Sequence Based Amplification
NS1	-	Nonstructural antigen 1
NT	-	Neutralization Test
PrM	-	Premembrane protein
PCR	-	Polymerase Chain Reaction

PCV	-	Packed Cell Volume
PLCE1	-	Phospholipase C epsilon 1 (An effector of Ras)
RNasin	-	Recombinant mammalian RNase inhibitor
RT-PCR	-	Reverse Transcriptase PCR
RT-LAMP	-	Reverse-Transcriptase Loop-Assisted-Isothermal-Amplification
SEAR	-	South East Asia Region
SDA	-	Strand Displacement Amplification
TNF	-	Tumour Necrosis Factor
TGF	-	Transforming Growth Factor

CHAPTER 1: INTRODUCTION

Dengue is a mosquito borne *flavivirus* infection found in tropical and subtropical regions of the world and threatens approximately half of the world population. The disease spectrum ranges from asymptomatic infection to moderate febrile illness (Dengue Fever) to more serious fatal haemorrhagic disease forms, Dengue Haemorrhagic Fever (DHF) and Dengue Shock Syndrome (DSS) [1-5]. Despite control measures, dengue continues to emerge with increased number of cases, severity, expansion to rural areas and newer geographies. The associated high morbidity poses threat to international travelers, military deployments and emanates a promising bioweapon potential. In the absence of licensed vaccines or specific antiviral therapy, patient management relies entirely on good supportive care.

Early, sensitive and specific diagnosis is paramount for patient management, prevention of complications, etiologic investigation and disease control. Early diagnosis is achieved by NS1 antigen detection, nucleic acid amplification and virus isolation. NS1 antigen detection through lateral flow immunochromatography (LF-ICT) is highly sensitive and specific but unable to identify serotype. Nucleic acid techniques such as reverse transcriptase polymerase chain reaction (RT-PCR), real time PCR and multiplex PCR (M-PCR) are highly sensitive and specific and able to identify serotypes, though require expensive equipments for amplification and detection of amplified products [6-9]. Nucleic acid based assays are emerging as the gold standard for the rapid diagnosis of dengue. Virus isolation needs sophisticated labs and is not used widely. Diagnosis after four days is conferred by IgM and IgG based serological techniques such as enzyme linked immunosorbent assay (ELISA), hemagglutination inhibition (HI), complement fixation (CF) and neutralization test (NT). IgM μ capture ELISA is simple and requires less equipments. HI is more sensitive although equally specific as IgM μ capture ELISA using paired serum samples. IgG ELISA is nonspecific and exhibits cross-reactivity among flaviviruses. Both IgM/IgG based immunoassays cannot identify serotypes [6, 7].

CHAPTER 2: ETYMOLOGY, HISTORY AND EPIDEMIOLOGY OF DENGUE

Etymology

The word "Dengue" comes from Swahili "Ka-Dinga pepo", describing it as a sudden cramp like disease caused by an evil spirit. Various names such as Breakbone fever, Breakheart fever, la dengue, Dandy Fever, Infectious Thrombocytopenic Purpura, Singapore/Thai/Philippine Haemorrhagic Fever have been given.

History of Dengue

Earliest reports of a dengue like disease are from Chin Dynasty China (265-420 A.D.). The first cases of DF were recorded almost simultaneously in Cairo and Alexandria (Egypt, 1799), Jakarta (Indonesia, 1799) and Philadelphia (United States, 1780). The virus was identified in the 1943 when it was causing a large number of non-combat casualties to allied and Japanese forces by Japanese scientists shortly followed by U.S. researchers. Four serotypes of the virus were identified by 1956 long before the discovery of fifth serotype which has been described recently [10].

Dengue has now become a leading public health problem worldwide and is a notifiable disease. Many outbreaks and epidemics of DF or DHF causing high morbidity and mortality during the past few decades have strained the tropical developing nation health system worldwide including Asia-Pacific, Africa, Americas and Eastern Mediterranean regions. World Health Organization (WHO) reported 10,000 laboratory confirmed cases in 1996 epidemic and 2185 cases in 2003 outbreak [2, 3, 4].

Epidemiology and World Picture

Dengue is endemic in 110 tropical and subtropical countries and threatens 2.5 billion (about 40%) of the world population [6]. Dengue was considered a sporadic disease causing epidemics at long intervals till World War II. Destruction of existing water systems and subsequent water storage during and after World War II contributed to habitat for *Aedes aegypti* larvae and facilitated the transport of mosquitoes and their eggs to new geographical areas [11-13]. International estimates indicate 100 million DF cases and 50 million DHF cases annually throughout the world with a case fatality of 0.5% to 3.5% in Asian counties. Disease burden is estimated to be 465,000 disability adjusted life years. DHF first emerged as a public health problem in 1954 during Manila epidemic and thereafter became a leading cause of hospitalization and death among children in South East Asia region (SEAR). Subsequently, dengue spread to Pacific islands and continental Americas by 1970s. Several epidemics by all four serotypes, predominantly DEN2, occurred in the world in 1980s and 1990s. The first major DHF epidemic in 1984 in Sri Lanka was followed by yearly increase in epidemics in SEAR including India, predominantly by DEN3 [14-16]. The 1998 dengue pandemic involved 56 countries worldwide. In 2005, Brazil and Americas reported over 390,000 and 609,000 DHF cases respectively, attributed to DEN3 [17] (Fig 1-3).

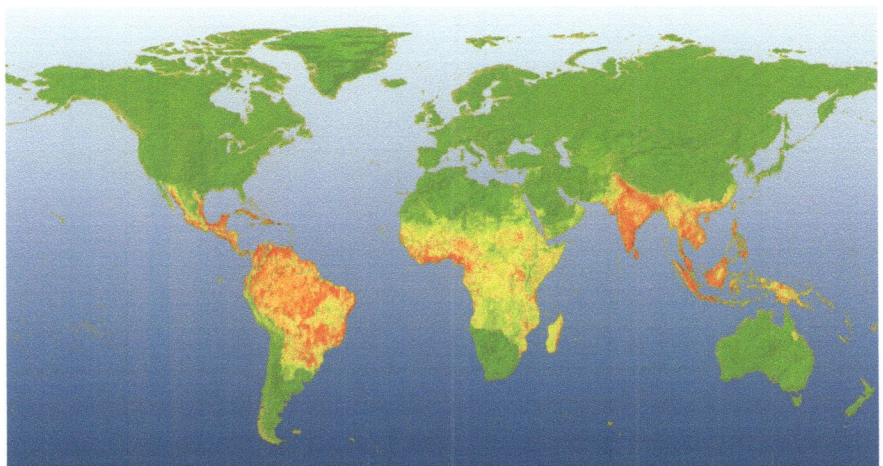

Fig 1: World distribution of Dengue
Source: CNN News article, "Study suggests new approach to dengue fever", Apr 7, 2013

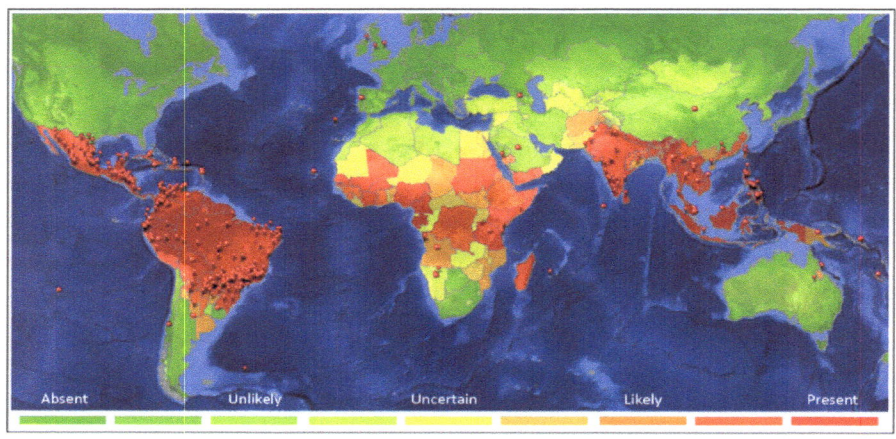

Fig 2: World distribution of Dengue severity

Source: www.healthmap.org

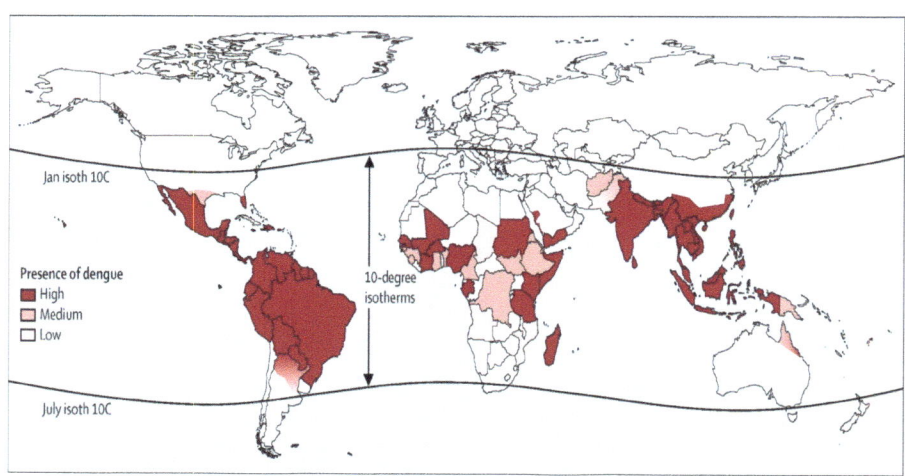

Fig 3: World distribution of Dengue

Source: Lancet: "Dengue", http://dx.doi.org/10.1016/S0140-6736(14)60572-9

Dengue in the Indian subcontinent

Since the first major epidemic at Kolkata in 1963, more than 80 outbreaks have been reported at regular intervals from different parts of the country except North East [18, 19]. Epidemics by all four serotypeswith increasing reports of hemorrhagic manifestations have been reported from Maharashtra, Gujarat, Rajasthan, Karnataka, Punjab and Uttar Pradesh [19-23]. Outbreaks of DF/DHF have been reported in Delhi during years 1967, 1970, 1982, 1988, 1992 and 1996 by DEN1 and DEN2, although DEN3 and DEN4 have also been reported. The 1996 DHF outbreak in Delhi and surrounding states caused by DEN2 lead to more than 10252 hospitalizations and 423 deaths [20]. Delhi and adjoining areas were again struck by a major outbreak of DF/DHF in 2009, predominantly by DEN3 [2, 4].

CHAPTER 3: VIROLOGY OF DENGUE

Structure and genome of Dengue Virus

Dengue is an enveloped nucleocapsid spherical virus, about 40-50 nm in diameter with particles of 7 nm on its surface. It is a positive stranded RNA flavivirus, belonging to the family *Flaviviridae* and genus *Flavivirus*. There are five serotypes (DEN1, DEN2, DEN3, DEN4 and DEN5) classified according to biological and immunological criteria [5]. The mature virus contains a single stranded, positive sense RNA genome of approximately 10200 Kb, coding for three structured proteins (capsid C, pre-membrane PrM and envelope E) and seven nonstructural proteins (NS1, NS2a, NS2b, NS3, NS4a, NS4b and NS5). The gene order is 5'-C-prM (M)-E-NS1-NS2A-NS2B-NS3-NS4A-NS4B-NS5-3', as for other flaviviruses (Fig 4-5). The virus genome with a large openreading frame encodes a polyprotein precursor of about 3000 amino acids that are processed cotranslationally andposttranslationally by viral and host proteases [24]. The structural proteins derived from the polyprotein precursor are included in the mature virion, whereas NS proteins play various roles in virus replication and polypeptide processing [25].

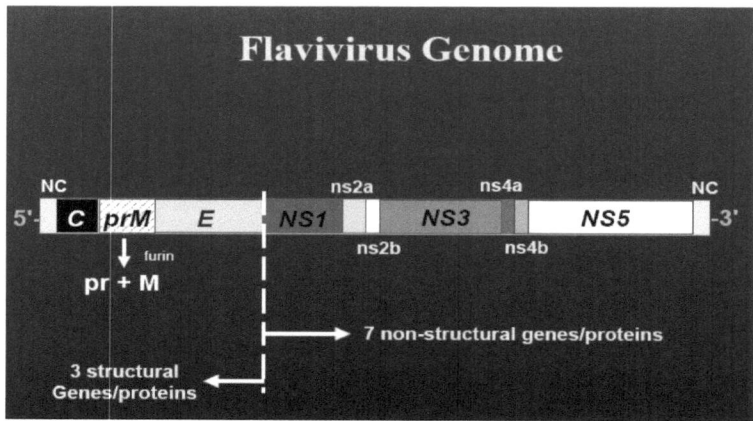

Fig 4: Dengue virus genome

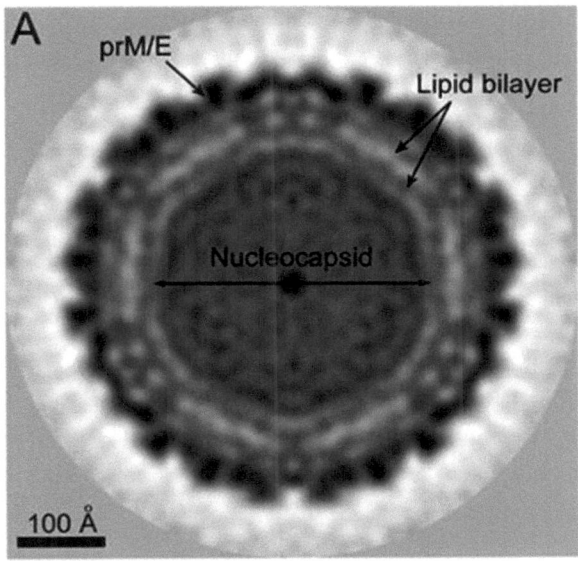

Fig 5: Dengue virus structure

Source: Purdue University, http://www.purdue.edu/uns/x/2008a/080327RossmannMature.html

Translational genomics of Dengue

Nonstructural proteins, expressed as both membrane-associated and secreted forms have been implicated in the pathogenesis of severe disease. Plasma levels of secreted NS1 are higher in patients with DHF compared to DF. Moreover, elevated free secreted NS1 levels within 72 hours of illness identify patients at risk of DHF [26].

The E glycoprotein contains antigenic determinants for hemagglutination and neutralization and is also predicted to be involved in the phenomenon of antibody dependent enhancement (ADE). It has been hypothesized that one of the important primary determinants of DHF reside in the amino acid 390 of E protein, which purportedly alters virion binding to host cells. The serotypes of dengue virus have been classified into the genotypes on the basis of the variations found in the nucleotide sequence of E protein.

The C protein interacts with RNA to form the virion nucleocapsid. The dengue C protein is essential in virus assembly to ensure specific encapsidation of the viral genome.

The prM glycoprotein regulates polymerization of E protein [14].

Serotypes

Five distinct but antigenically related serotypes; DEN1-5 are prevalent in the tropical developing world. Multiple sequential infections with different serotypes are possible in hyperendemic regions as primary dengue infection induces serotype specific immunity. Secondary infection is a major risk factor for DHF and DSS through antibody dependent enhancement [5]. Epidemics of DHF/DSS rapidly strain the developing nation health system. Lifelong immunity conferred is serotype specific without any cross protective immunity for other serotypes. A person can be infected by all four serotypes in a lifetime [27-28].

Genotypes

Three genotypes have been defined for DEN1, five for DEN2, four for DEN3 and two for DEN4. Each genotype seems to have a defined focus of endemicity. The difference in virulence of different strains is attributable to variation in genotypes. A new genotype replacing an earlier circulating strain may result in a severe form of dengue [27-28]. The dengue serotypes share antigenic epitopes with other serotypes as well as other *Flaviviruses* interfering with serological diagnosis.

CHAPTER 4: DENGUE VECTORS AND TRANSMISSION

Dengue is transmitted from viremic to susceptible humans through mosquitoes belonging to the genus *Aedes* and subgenus *Stegomyia* (Fig 6). *Aedes aegypti* is the most important epidemic vector, but other species such as *A. albopictus*, *A. polynesiensis*, *A. scutellaris* complex and *A. niveus* may act as vectors depending on the geographical location. *Aedes albopictus* has been found to transmit dengue in India, Thailand, Samui Island, Singapore and Mexico [6]. (Fig 7)

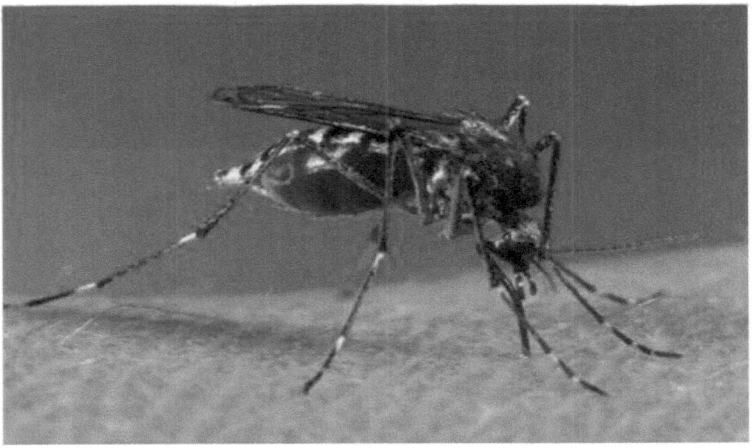

Fig 6: *Aedes* mosquito
Source: Google images, free web content

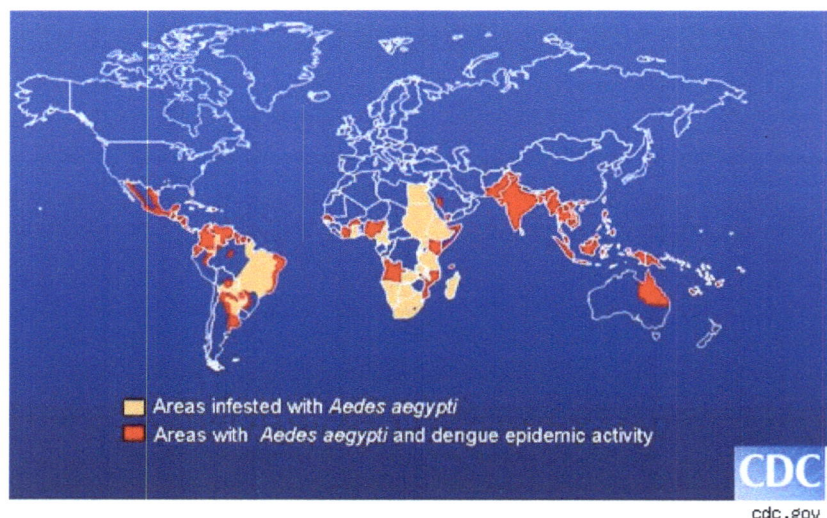

Fig 7: World distribution of *Aedes* mosquito
Source: CDC, Atlanta

Epidemic Vector

Aedes aegypti (Tiger mosquito), is a small, black and white, highly domesticated tropical mosquito that prefers to lay its eggs in artificial containers commonly found in and around homes, e.g. flower vases, automobile tyres, buckets and trash. Its eggs can withstand dessication for about a year making dengue eradication difficult. The adult female mosquitoes rest indoors, are unobtrusive and are very nervous daytime feeders. (Fig 8)

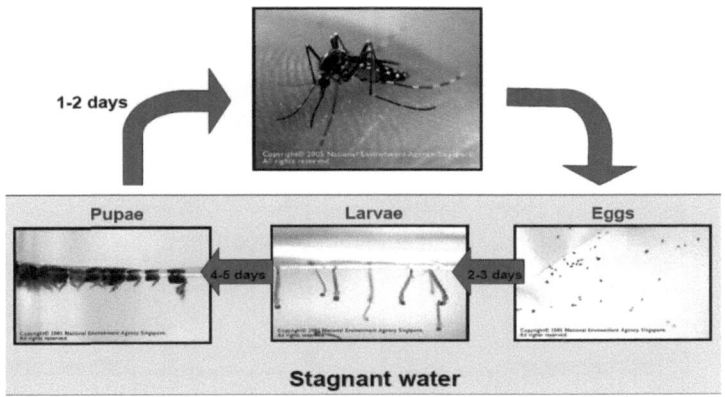

Fig 8: Life cycle of *Aedes* mosquito
Source: http://alrazaak.com/threads/140-What-is-Dengue-Fever-Signs-Symptoms-Stages-Treatment#.WBt9V8k-bIU

Transmission of Dengue

The mosquito acquires infection from viremic feeds during febrile episodes. Dengue virus replicates in the mid gut, reaches the haemocoel and haemolymph, gains access to different tissues of the insect and reaches the salivary glands in 8-10 days (extrinsic incubation period) rendering the mosquito infective for its lifetime (2-4 weeks) (Fig 9). Transovarian (vertical) and sexual transmission is known [29, 30]. Man to man transmission by intrapartum, percutaneous and mucocutaneous routes has been reported [31]. DF/DHF occurs predominantly among urban populations where density of dwellings and short flying distance of the vector create the right conditions for transmission. Rural epidemics have also been reported and are attributed to transport contact, mobility and spread of peri-urbanisation [32-36]. Dengue epidemics have been associated with rainy season [36]. In India, post monsoon season marks the onset of dengue reaching a peak in September to November and ending with the onset of winter.

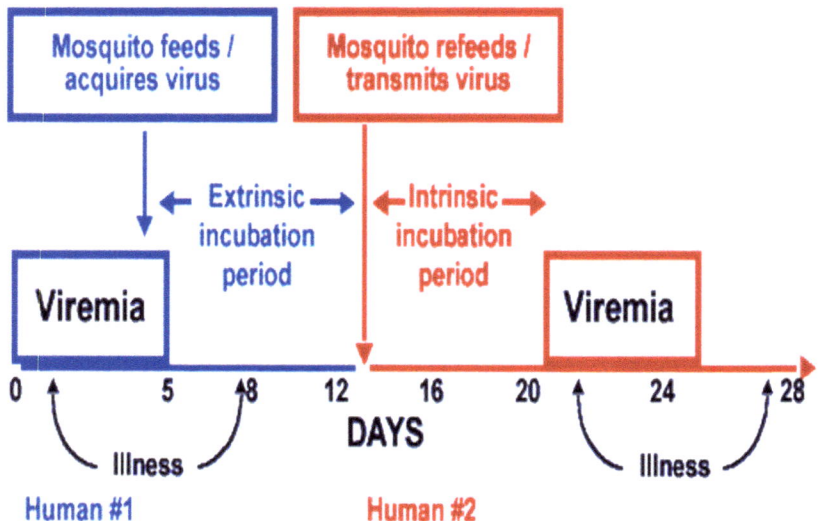

Fig 9: Incubation period of Dengue

CHAPTER 5: DENGUE VIRAL INFECTION AND HOST FACTORS

Dengue Viral infection

Dengue virus binds to its receptor mediated by E protein after which it is fused into acidic lysosomes through receptor-mediated endocytosis [37]. Dengue virus enters Langerhans cells of skin through binding between viral proteins and membrane proteins, specifically the C-type lectins such as DC-SIGN/L-SIGN, mannose receptor, heparan sulfate, nLc4Cer and CLEC5A. DEN-2 also binds with HSP70/HSP90, GRP78, CD14-associated protein and two unknown proteins having trypsin resistance and trypsin sensitive properties. DEN1–3 serotypes bind with Laminin receptor while DEN2–4 serotypes bind with an unknown protein as well [24, 38, 39]. The virus genome is translated in membrane bound vesicles on endoplasmic reticulum and new viral proteins replicate viral RNA. Immature virus particles are transported to Golgi apparatus and get released by exocytosis through budding on maturation and infect monocytes and macrophages subsequently. In only few hours after infection, thousands of copies of viral molecules are produced from a single viral molecule leading to cell damage. Viral-encoded RNA-dependent RNA polymerases and other cellular factors are responsible for catalyzing the infection cycle of dengue virus [24]. The viral titres peak around the onset of clinical features, a time when the infection is widespread.

Host Factors

DF is an important cause of pediatric hospitalization in SEAR. Since 1980s, studies have reported a higher association of DHF with older ages [24, 32, 45, 51]. From 1990–96, the highest age-specific morbidity rates were in the 15 to 34 year age group. Males are commonly infected, although females are prone to severe disease possibly due to accelerated immune response [40-42]. Severe dengue has been observed less frequently in dengue infected black persons than whites [25]. Genetic polymorphisms increasing dengue risk include polymorphisms in genes coding for TNFα, mannan binding lectin, CTLA4, TGFβ, DC-SIGN, PLCE1, HLA-B and G6PD deficiency. Polymorphisms in the genes for the vitamin D receptor and FcγR are protective in secondary dengue infection [38, 43].

CHAPTER 6: IMMUNOLOGICAL RESPONSE TO DENGUE

Immunological Response

The virus is present in serum, plasma, peripheral blood mononuclear cells for a very short period. The acquired immune response to dengue infection consists of the production of IgM, IgG and IgA, specific for E protein. Detectable levels of anti-dengue antibodies appear few days after fever, leading to two types of responses, primary and secondary.

Primary Immunological Response

A person previously not infected with *flaviviruses* (e.g. yellow fever, Japanese encephalitis, tick born encephalitis) or immunized against them, mounts a primary antibody response wherein IgM appears first, rises rapidly and peaks at about 2 weeks after onset of symptoms and declines by 2-3 months. IgG appears in low titers at the end of first week, increases slowly peaking at 2 weeks and declining by 3-6 months. Both IgM and IgG antibodies neutralize dengue virus [1, 6, 7]. The physiological definition of primary dengue infection is characterized by high molar concentration of IgM antibodies and low IgG.

Secondary Immunological Response

Individuals with immunity due to previous *flavivirus* infection have pre-existing IgG antibodies which may persist for life (as measured by E/M antigen-coated indirect IgG ELISA). Many B-cell clones responding to the first flavivirus infection are restimulated to synthesize early antibody with a greater affinity for the first infecting virus than for the present infecting virus in every subsequent flavivirus infection. They may also mount a secondary anamnestic IgG antibody response characterized by rapid rise in IgG antibodies by 4-5 days of illness [44]. IgG antibodies have high degrees of cross-reactivity to homologous and heterologous flavivirus antigens. A small percentage of patients with secondary infections have no detectable IgM [45].

Secondary infection is responsible for most of the cases of DHF. In Dengue fever, IgA antibodies appear only between 8-11 days after onset of fever, whereas in DHF and DSS, IgA is undetectable in acute phase but increased in convalescent phase [46].

Antibody Dependent Enhancement

The 4 subtypes of different strains of dengue virus have 60-80% homology between each other. The immune response produces specific antibodies to that subtype's surface proteins that prevent the virus from binding to macrophage cells and gaining entry. However, if another subtype of dengue virus infects the individual, the virus will activate the immune system to attack it as if it was the first subtype. The antibodies bind to the surface proteins but do not inactivate the virus. The immune response attracts numerous macrophages in which the antigen-antibody complex is bound and internalized by immunoglobulin Fc receptors on the cell membrane of macrophages; but due to heterologous nature of antibodies, the virus is not neutralized and freely replicates inside the macrophages. This phenomenon is referred to as Antibody Dependent Enhancement (ADE) and is supported by epidemiological observations [47, 48].

This hypothesis implies that patients experiencing a second infection with a heterologous dengue serotype have a significantly higher risk for developing DHF [47-49]. The infected mononuclear cells produce and secrete vasoactive mediators (cytokines) in response to dengue infection, which causes increased vascular permeability leading to hypovolemia and shock [49, 50] (Fig 10-12).

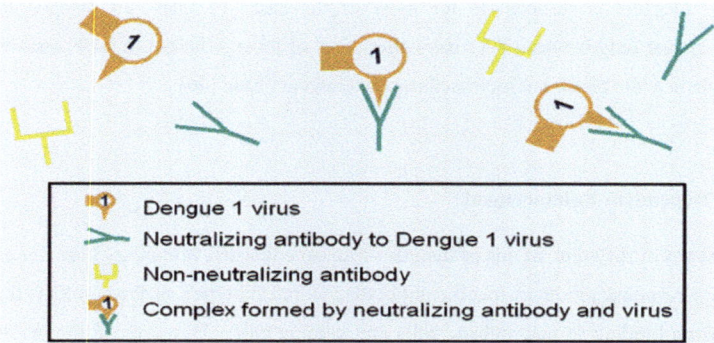

Fig 10: Depiction of homologous antibodies in primary infection

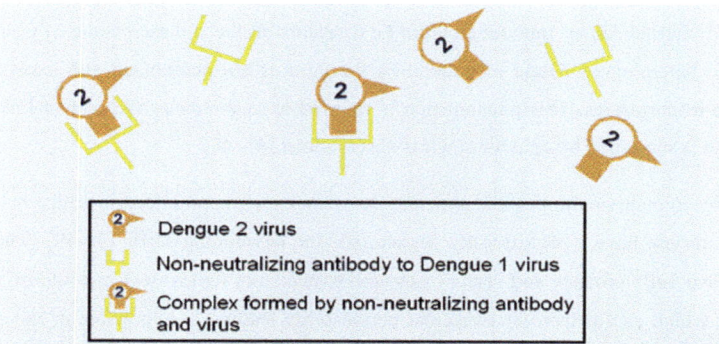

Fig 11: Depiction of non-neutralizing heterologous antibodies in secondary infection with a different serotype

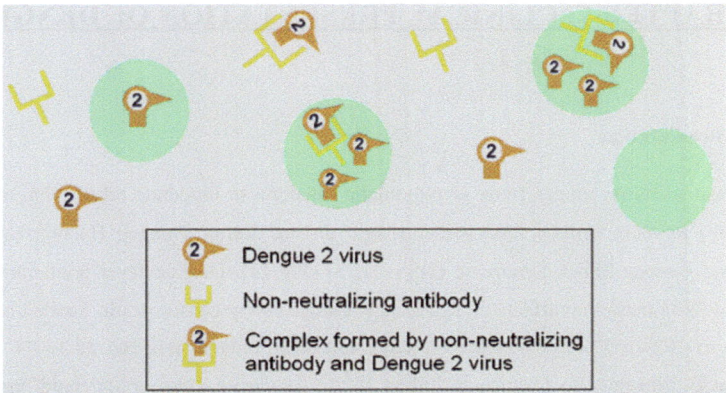

Fig 12: Depiction of invasion of monocytes by virus-antibody complexes which lead to the secretions of cytokines (Antibody dependent enhancement)

Secondary Dengue Infection

The dengue virus also infects CD4+ and CD8+ T cells. Following primary infection, both serotype specific and serotype cross reactive memory T cells are formed. On secondary exposure to the virus, more serotypes cross reactive CD4+ and CD8+ T-cells augment infection by producing interferon (IFN)-γ, TNF-α and TNF-β [51]. Virus upon infection activates IFN signalling pathway but dengue develops IFN resistance. NS2a, NS4a and NS4b block the IFN cascade to escape the immune response. NS4b inhibits IFN cascade by blocking STAT-1 phosphorylation [24].

Both qualitative and quantitative platelet defects develop and haemorrhage may not correlate with thrombocytopenia [5, 52]. There is focal necrosis of hepatocytes, swelling, appearance of Councilman Bodies and hyaline necrosis of Kupffer cells. Isolation of dengue virus from the brain and cerebrospinal fluid and intrathecal antibody production suggest dengue virus capable of crossing the blood-brain barrier [53, 54].

CHAPTER 7: CLINICAL PRESENTATION OF DENGUE

Clinical Presentation

The disease spectrum ranges from asymptomatic infection to moderate febrile illness (Dengue Fever; DF) to more serious fatal haemorrhagic disease forms, Dengue Haemorrhagic Fever (DHF) and Dengue Shock Syndrome (DSS) [1, 5] (Fig 13). Dengue fever is characterized by severe flu like illness that affects all age groups though rarely causes death. Sudden onset fever may rise to 102^0-105^0 F, persist for 2-7 days and drop, only to rebound 12 to 24 hour later (saddleback). Nonspecific features including frontal headache, retro-orbital pain, body aches, nausea and vomiting, joint pains, weakness, rash, anorexia, altered taste and throat pain are seen. Facial flushing or erythematous mottling occurring with fever may be followed by a second maculopapular rash beginning on the trunk and spreading to face and extremities between 2nd-4th day. Although, hemorrhagic manifestations are uncommon in dengue fever, petechiae, purpura, gastrointestinal bleeding, epistaxis and gingival bleeding may be observed in some individuals. Petechiae appear at end of the febrile phase and may be followed by intense pruritus or desquamation. Unusual features such as encephalitis, acalculus cholecystitis, fulminant hepatitis, severe vomiting or diarrhea may be seen. Recovery from dengue fever is uneventful but may be prolonged especially in adults [19, 55, 56]. WHO supports two case definitions from 1997 and 2009.

Case definition of dengue fever: (WHO 1997/2006) [6] (Fig 13)

Clinical description: An acute febrile illness of 2-7 days with 2 or more of the following: headache, retro-orbital or ocular pain, myalgia, arthralgia, rash, leucopenia and hemorrhagic manifestations (e.g., positive tourniquet test, petechiae, purpura/ecchymosis, epistaxis, gum bleeding, blood in vomit/urine/stool, vaginal bleeding).

Laboratory criteria for diagnosis: One or more of the following:

- Isolation of the dengue virus from serum, plasma, leukocytes, or autopsy samples,
- Demonstration of a four-fold or greater change in reciprocal IgG or IgM antibody titres to one or more dengue virus antigens in paired serum samples,
- Demonstration of dengue virus antigen in autopsy tissue by immunohistochemistry or immunofluorescence or in serum samples by ELISA,
- Detection of viral genomic sequences in autopsy tissue, serum or cerebrospinal fluid samples by PCR.

Case classification:

Suspected: A case compatible with the clinical description.

Probable: A case compatible with clinical description with one or more of the following:

- supportive serology (reciprocal HI antibody titre > 1280, comparable IgG ELISA titre or positive IgM antibody test in late acute or convalescent phase serum specimen), or
- Occurrence at same location and time as other confirmed cases of dengue fever

Confirmed: A case compatible with the clinical description, laboratory confirmed.

Reportable: Any probable or confirmed case should be reported

Case definition of dengue hemorrhagic fever (DHF): (WHO 1997/2006) [6]

A probable or confirmed case of dengue and hemorrhagic tendencies evidenced by one or more of the following:

1. Fever lasting from 2-7 days, occasionally biphasic
2. Positive tourniquet test
3. Petechiae, ecchymoses or purpura
4. Bleeding: mucosa, gastrointestinal tract, injection sites or other sites

5. Haematemesis or malaena

and thrombocytopenia (100 000/mm^3 cells or less)

and evidence of plasma leakage due to increased vascular permeability, manifested by one or more of the following:

6. more than 20% rise in average hematocrit for age and sex
7. more than 20% drop in hematocrit following volume replacement compared to baseline
8. signs of plasma leakage (pleural effusion, ascites, hypoproteinemia)

Case definition of dengue shock syndrome (DSS): (WHO 1997/2006) [6]

All the above criteria for DHF plus evidence of circulatory failure manifested by (1) rapid and weak pulse and (2) narrow pulse pressure (<20 mm Hg/2.7 kPa) or (a) Hypotension for age (b) Cold, clammy skin, restlessness and altered mental status [5, 11].

Laboratory criteria for DHF/DSS: One or more of the following:

- Rapidly developing, severe thrombocytopenia (i.e., <100,000 cells/mm^3 [<100 x 10^9/L])
- Decreased total WCC and neutrophils and changing neutrophil-to-lymphocyte ratio
- Elevated haematocrit (i.e., 20% increase from baseline is objective evidence of plasma leakage)
- Hypoalbuminaemia (i.e., serum albumin <35 g/L [3.5 g/dL] suggests plasma leakage)
- Elevated LFTs (i.e., AST:ALT >2) (Fig 13)

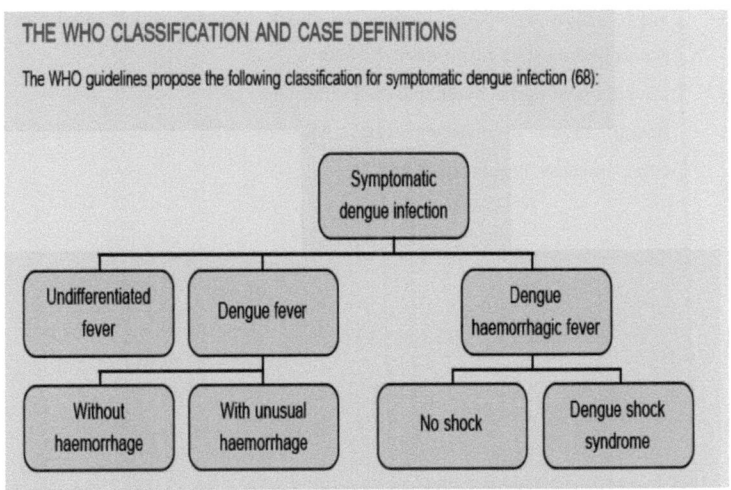

Fig 13: WHO Classification and Case Definitions

Case definition of dengue fever: (WHO 2009) (Fig 14)

Dengue without warning signs

Fever with any two from nausea/vomiting, rash, aches and pains, leucopenia and positive tourniquet test.

Dengue with warning signs

Dengue as defined above with any one from abdominal pain or tenderness, persistent vomiting, clinical fluid accumulation (ascites, pleural effusion), mucosal bleeding, lethargy/restlessness, liver enlargement >2 cm, increased hematocrit concurrent with rapid decrease in platelet count.

Severe Dengue

Dengue as defined above with any one from the following

a) Severe plasma leakage leading to shock (dengue shock syndrome) or fluid accumulation with respiratory distress
b) Severe bleeding (as evaluated by a clinician)
c) Severe organ involvement (i.e., AST or ALT 1000 or greater, impaired consciousness, organ failure).

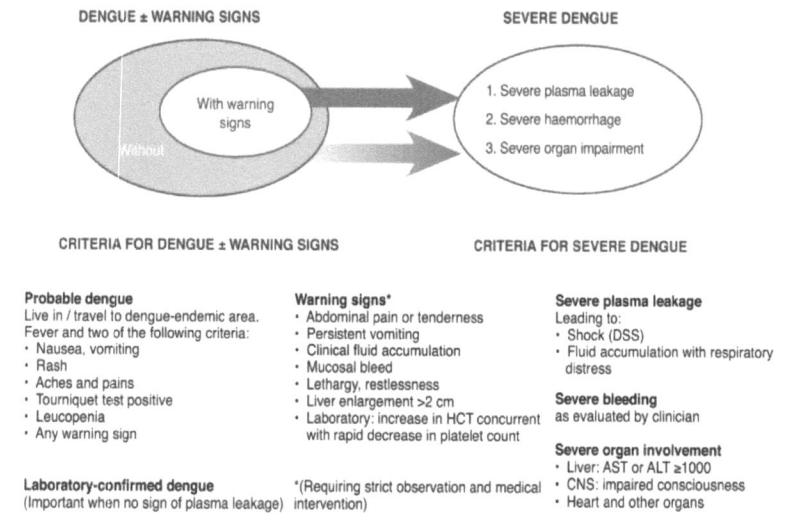

Fig 14: WHO Classification and Case Definitions 2009

Dengue Hemorrhagic Fever and Dengue Shock Syndrome

DHF is primarily a disease of children under the age of 15 years although it may also occur in adults [5]. DHF usually follows secondary dengue infections, but may sometimes follow primary infections especially in infants. DHF is characterized by four major clinical manifestations i.e. high grade fever, hemorrhagic phenomenon, hepatomegaly and features of circulatory failure. The major pathophysiological change differentiating DHF from DF is an acute increase in vascular permeability leading to plasma leakage evidenced by serous effusion found post mortem, pleural effusion on X-ray, hemoconcentration (>20% reduction in plasma volume) and hypoproteinemia. Bleeding time can be prolonged even with platelet counts above $100,000/mm^3$. The presence of thrombocytopenia with concurrent hemoconcentration differentiates DHF from DF.

The critical stage in DHF is the time of defervescence, but signs of circulatory failure or hemorrhagic manifestations may occur from about 24 hrs before to 24 hrs after the temperature falls to normal or below. Fever lasts for 2-7 days and is followed by a fall in the temperature to normal or sub normal levels. At this point the patient may recover or progress to the phase of plasma leakage. Those who remain ill despite their temperature subsiding are more likely to progress to DSS. This afebrile phase is the critical stage of the disease. A rapid fall in temperature is often accompanied by tachycardia and hypotension. Many patients recover spontaneously or after a short period of fluid and electrolyte therapy. In severe cases, shock ensues and can progress rapidly to profound shock and death. Common hemorrhagic manifestations include positive tourniquet test, skin hemorrhages such as petechiae, purpuric lesions and ecchymosis. Epistaxis, bleeding gums, gastrointestinal hemorrhage and haematuria occur less frequently. Vaginal bleeding is commonly seen in females. Convalescence in DHF is usually short and uneventful [5, 11, 19].

Differential Diagnosis of Dengue Fever and DHF

The differential diagnosis associated with DF and DHF include a wide variety of viral (West Nile fever, Japanese Encephalitis, Chikungunya), bacteria (typhoid, meningococcal septicemia), spirochetes (leptospirosis), parasitic (malaria) and rickettsial infection that produce a similar syndrome. Chikungunya and malaria is endemic in many parts of country and peak season of disease transmission coincides with dengue [5, 11]. Due to epidemiological similarities it is not unusual to experience concurrent epidemic of dengue infection with other infection, such as leptospirosis, typhoid fever and malaria [55, 57]. Concurrent infections by multiple dengue serotypes has been reported [54].

CHAPTER 8: LABORATORY DIAGNOSIS OF DENGUE

Laboratory Diagnosis

Laboratory diagnosis can be achieved by detection of NS1 antigen, IgM, IgG and IgA antibodies, culture of the virus and nucleic acid amplification. Blood, serum, plasma, washed leucocytes, cerebrospinal fluid, saliva, tissues can be used. Multiple and sequential flavivirus infections make differential diagnosis difficult due to the presence of preexisting antibodies, original antigenic sin (flaviviruses) and anamnestic IgG antibody response (dengue virus) in regions where many flaviviruses/many dengue virus serotypes are co-circulating.

Antigen detection

ELISA and dot-blot assays demonstrating high concentrations of the E/M antigens and NS1 antigen in the form of immune complexes, can be detected in acute phase sera. NS1 antigen is a valuable surrogate marker for viremia in the initial 12-48 hrs of infection. It can be detected by lateral flow immunochromatography (LF-ICT), NS1 capture ELISA, immunofluorescence assay (IFA), microsphere based immunoassay, dot-blot assay, immunochemistry, immunoperoxidase and avidin-biotin enzyme assays. Type-specific monoclonal antibody immunofluorescence staining may identify dengue serotypes.

Immunochromatography

LF-ICT is a simple and rapid test with 100% sensitivity, high specificity and usefulfor mass screening [8]. Pre-existing virus-IgG complexes may interfere in acute stage of secondary infections.

NS1 capture ELISA

Serotype specific monoclonal antibody based NS1 antigen capture ELISA can differentiate primary and secondary dengue infections.

IFA

IFA can be performed with infected cell cultures, mosquito brain, tissue squashes, mouse brain squashes or even on formalin fixed tissues embedded in paraffin and sectioned for histopathologic testing. Serotype specific monoclonal antibodies produced in tissue culture or mouse ascitic fluids and an anti-mouse immunoglobulin G-fluorescein isothiocyanate conjugate are used. Multiple viruses in patients with concurrent infections with more than one serotype can be detected [39, 57].

Immunohistochemistry

Dengue antigens can be visualized in tissue sections using labeled monoclonal/polyclonal antibodies that are visualized with markers such as fluorescent dyes, enzyme conjugates (peroxidase, phosphatase) or colloidal gold.

Antibody detection

Various serological tests such as LF-ICT, particle agglutination, IgM μ capture ELISA, indirect IgG ELISA, hemagglutination-inhibition (HI), complement fixation (CFT), neutralization test (NT), microsphere based immunoassay, indirect immunofluorescent antibody test, microneutralisation assay, dot-blot assay and Western Blot assay can be used for detection of IgM and IgG. IgA and IgE antibodies have also been evaluated and found to be useful in secondary infections [36]. Unequivocal serologic diagnosis depends upon a significant (four-fold or greater) rise in the titer of specific antibodies between acute and convalescent phase serum samples. An IgM/IgG ratio < 1.2 indicates secondary infection [36]. Rapid test kits are based on

LF-ICT or particle agglutination. LF-ICT can detect NS1, IgM and IgG in one test and rapidly differentiate primary and secondary dengue infections [8].

Enzyme linked immunosorbent assay (ELISA)

ELISA under various formats has been used such as E/M specific IgM μ capture ELISA, NS1 serotype specific IgG ELISA, Pathozyme IgM/IgG, Platelia Dengue NS1 antigen ELISA, IgG avidity ELISA, capture ultramicro ELISA, Dot ELISA and AuBioDOT IgM capture. IgM μ capture ELISA is simple, rapid, requires minimal equipment and hence widely used. Single dilution, non quantitative test on a properly timed single blood sample may indicate recent *flavivirus* infection including dengue. It is less sensitive but as specific as HI. Monotypic response may be observed specific to dengue though not amongst serotypes [45, 58]. ELISA is an invaluable tool for surveillance of DF and DHF/DSS in endemic areas and random population based surveys and viral illness in areas where dengue is not endemic. Indirect IgG ELISA and IgG avidity ELISA is simple and easy to perform and can be used to differentiate primary and secondary dengue infection. Avidity of IgG is low after primary antigenic challenge but matures slowly within weeks and months after infection [59].

Haemagglutination inhibition test (HI)

HI is sensitive, easy to perform and requires minimal equipment. HI antibodies begin to appear at detectable levels (titer of 10) by day 5-6 of illness, peak at 1:640 in primary infections whereas titres of 1:1280 or greater are common in secondary infections [45]. HI antibodies persist for long periods (up to 48 years and probably longer). By contrast, there is an immediate anamnestic response in secondary dengue infections, and reciprocal antibody titers increase rapidly within few days of illness, often reaching 5120-10240 or more. Such high levels of HI antibody fall below 1280 by 30-40 days, though may persist for 2-3 months in some patients [45]. HI test is suitable for seroepidemiologic studies, butnot suitable for secondary infections. It is unable to identify serotypes, however, some patients with primary infections show a relatively monotypic HI response that generally correlates with the virus isolated [45, 58].

Complement Fixation Test (CFT)

CFT is based on the principle that complement is consumed during antigen-antibody reactions. Complement fixation antibodies generally appear later than HI antibodies, are more specific in primary infections and usually persist for short periods, although low levels of antibodies persist in some persons. It is neither specific in secondary infections nor suitable for seroepidemiologic studies. CFT is also exacting in time and effort and not widely used.

Neutralization test (NT)

Serum dilution plaque reduction NT is sensitive and specific. Antibodies rise at about the same time as HI and ELISA but quicker than CFT and persist for up to 48 years. NT may be positive in the absence of detectable HI antibodies in some persons with past dengue infection and thus can be used for seroepidemiologic studies. NT can also be use for serotyping of dengue virus [36]. NT is exacting in time, effort and cost and not used routinely [45, 58, 60].

Molecular Detection

Molecular methods include Polymerase chain reaction (RT-PCR, real time PCR, nested PCR, in situ PCR, M-PCR), isothermal amplification techniques (Nucleic Acid Sequence Based Amplification, Self sustained sequence replication, Strand displacement amplification, Rolling circle amplification, reverse-transcriptase loop mediated isothermal amplification) and nucleic acid hybridization are useful in acute phase samples corresponding to viremia. They can be employed in various samples viz. sera, autopsy tissues, mosquito pool, mosquito larvae and infected cell cultures. The outcome of these tests is not influenced by the presence of neutralizing antibodies and thus they may be positive in convalescent phase samples as well [61]. They are also helpful for serotyping of the virus in a multiplexed format. The existing techniques are highly sensitive and specific. They can successfully augment existing methodologies and also work as reference tests.

However, they are sensitive to amplicon contamination and hence tests need to incorporate controls and results need to be interpreted in conjunction with virus isolation and serological tests. Molecular detection requires sophisticated instruments like thermal cycler for amplification and UV transilluminator for detection of amplified products on an agarose gel [61]. Their use is limited by acquisition capacity of resource limited laboratories, expertise and standardization [62-66]. More sensitive and real time based assays having the advantages of rapidity, quantitative measurement, lower contamination rate, higher sensitivity, higher specificity, and easy standardization. Real time nucleic acid amplification might eventually replace virus isolation and conventional RT-PCR as the new gold standard for the rapid diagnosis of virus infection.

Polymerase Chain Reaction

RT-PCR, utilizing consensus primers based on the conserved non-structural-3 gene, is simple, rapid, sensitive, reproducible and can detect viral RNA in clinical samples, autopsy tissues or mosquitoes, thereby enabling laboratory screening, entomological surveillance and molecular epidemiological studies [67, 68]. Lanciotti *et al.* developed a two-step nested RT-PCR test to amplify a 511 bp fragment using consensual primers, designed to amplify the C and prM genes of dengue viruses. The two step nested RT-PCR requires 13-14 hrs for complete serotypic characterization, and thus cannot produce the results on the same day. Real time RT-PCR is rapid, fully automated, single tube assay having the ability to provide quantitative measurements, lower contamination rate, higher sensitivity and specificity and easy standardization. Amplification is detected directly by monitoring fluorescence intensity obtained from fluorescent dyes linked to oligonucleotide probes which bind to amplified products. Five main chemical formats (the DNA binding fluorophores, the 5_nuclease, adjacent linear and hairpin oligonucleotide probes, and self-fluorescing amplicons) are used to detect the PCR product during real-time PCR [69]. The most widely used format is the 5-33-nuclease oligonucleotide probes (TaqMan assay) which is highly specific due to the sequence-specific hybridization of the probe [70]. M-PCR utilizes consensus forward dengue primer (D1) and four reverse primers TS1, TS2, TS3 and TS4 belonging to DEN 1-4 serotypes in a single PCR tube [71, 72]. *In situ* PCR can be carried out on tissue slides [59]. PCR is sensitive and specific, but limited by requirement of time, expertise, high precision instruments for amplification/detection of amplification and inability to identify genotypes.

Isothermal amplification techniques

Nucleic Acid Sequence Based Amplification (NASBA) is an RNA amplification technique that utilizes the action of avian myeloblastosis-reverse transcriptase (AMV-RT), T7-RNA polymerase and RNAse-H and detects amplification products by electrochemilumiescence (ECL). Studies have shown NASBA as 98.5% sensitive and 100% specific when compared to viral isolation from the C6/36 cell line for diagnosing dengue [33]. Isothermal amplification methods like NASBA, Self-sustained Sequence Replication and Rolling Circle Amplification can detect less than 10 copies within an hour but are compromised in specificity due to low stringency (40^0C) leading to poor target sequence selection and therefore not suitable as diagnostic tests. Strand displacement amplification (SDA) largely overcomes these shortcomings by using four primers but has increased backgrounds due to digestion, irrelevant DNA contained in the sample and the necessity to use costly nucleotides as a substrate. Multiple primers in SDA have improved amplification specificity for the target sequence although residual co-amplification of irrelevant sequences still causes a general setback in nucleic acid amplification, particularly for diagnostic use.

RT-LAMP is based on the principle of a strand displacement reaction and stem-loop structure. It is rapid, efficient, cost effective and highly specific. Six primers recognizing eight distinct sequences of the target in a single tube with *Bst* DNA polymerase at 63°C, produce 10^9 copies within an hour. Detection of amplification can be done by agarose gel electrophoresis, turbidimetry, UV lamp and even by naked eye visualization of magnesium pyrophosphate [70].

Hybridization probes

The hybridization probe method detects viral nucleic acids with cloned hybridization probes of variable specificity ranging from dengue complex to serotype specific. The method is rapid, simple and can be used on both clinical and postmortem samples. Hybridization combined with

RT-PCR may enhance sensitivity and specificity as hybridization probes have limited sensitivity. RT-PCR products labeled with digoxigenin may be hybridized with individual biotinylated type-specific PCR primers acting as capture probes immobilized on solid phase via streptavidin-coated tubes. The hybridized RT-PCR products can be quantitated spectrophotometrically via anti-digoxigenin antibodies conjugated with an enzyme which reacts with colorimetric substrate using an ELISA reader [74]. The difficulties of working with RNA and the technical expertise required to obtain reproducible results make this method more suitable as a research tool than as a routine diagnostic test [67].

Virus culture

Various isolation systems may be used for dengue viruses such as mammalian cell cultures, mosquito cell lines, intrathoracic inoculation of adult mosquitoes and intracerebral inoculation of 1-3 day old suckling mice. Mosquito inoculation combined with immunofluorescence is the most sensitive method especially in fatal DHF/DSS cases and wild viruseswith isolation rates of up to 100% [45, 58, 75]. Many endemic dengue virus strains can be recovered only by this method. The maintenance of an insectary limits its widespread use [74]. Both male and female mosquito cell lines from *Aedes albopictus* (C6/36 clone), *Aedes pseudoscutellaris* (AP61, AP64), *A. aegypti*, *A. krombeini*, *Toxorhynchites splendensa* and *T. amboinensis* have been used. Other cell lines such as Tra-284 and CLA1 have been used. Dengue viruses replicate in 4-5 days. Virus detection in mosquito cell linesis generally performed by the direct fluorescent antibody (DFA) test on mosquito brain or salivary glands [45]. Risk of laboratory infectionsis reduced by using male *Aedes* or nonbiting *Toxorhynchites* species [45, 60, 75]. Mammalian cell cultures (LLC-MK2, Vero) and mice are expensive, slow and insensitive. Inoculation in baby mice is very insensitive often requiring serial blind passages to allow adaptation to the virus and many wild type viruses cannot be isolated. Viruses require many passages before a consistent cytopathic effect can be observed [45, 75]. Viral culture is laborious, time consuming, expensive, has low sensitivity and cannot be widely used.

Immune Electron Microscopy

It aids rapid diagnosis and eliminates the need of specific reagents. However, it is not suitable for large tissues, requires high viral titres in liquids and nonspecific structures resemble viruses creating confusion. It may be a useful adjunct to other methods.

CHAPTER 9: RAPID DIAGNOSIS IN EPIDEMIC SCENARIO

Choice of diagnostic test

Rapidity, sensitivity, specificity, suitability at a particular stage of disease, ease of execution, standardization and automation determine choice of the test. It is imperative to identify tests suitable in various stages of the disease so as to aid timely treatment, etiologic investigation, vector and disease control. Suitability in resource limited epidemic and outbreak settings is also important. Regions endemic for dengue and related viruses are overwhelmed by the sudden surge of cases during outbreaks. Resource limited facilities in regions endemic for dengue and other related viruses are often overwhelmed by the sudden surge of cases during outbreaks and find it difficult to justify diagnosis of every dengue case using the WHO criteria or be able to differentiate it from other concurrent viral illnesses. Most resource limited facilities tend to diagnose and treat dengue based on similar clinical presentation during outbreaks. Related mosquito transmitted co-endemic viral illnesses such as Japanese Encephalitis, West Nile Fever, Yellow Fever, Chikungunya Fever may create considerable interference with diagnosis of dengue.

Rapid diagnosis of dengue

Rapid laboratory diagnosis of dengue infection is important to implement therapy, monitor prognosis and prevent complications such as DHF and DSS. Acute dengue infection is characterized by viremia which can be detected by NS1 antigen detection and RT-PCR [75, 76, 77]. Usually IgM and IgG antibodies start appearing in the serum after 5th day of acute dengue infection. RT-PCR is positive in the first five days of illness when the dengue serology is negative [74, 76, 77]. NS1 and IgM may be positive with early seroconvert patient where NS1 is declining and IgM/IgG antibodies have started to rise, sometimes representing inadequacy of the test to differentiate between acute and convalescent phase of dengue. Though, RT-PCR is a marker of dengue viremia seen in the acute phase, it may be positive in the convalescent phase owing to incomplete neutralization of the virus and persistence of dead/fragmented viral nucleic acid. Samples positive either for IgM antibodies alone or both IgM and IgG antibodies may form a complex with viral particles and cause hindrance in viral detection [9].

Combined antigen-antibody testing

NS1 antigen and molecular methods are the most reliable diagnostic tests for early detection of dengue when the viral titres are at their peak level. IgM antibodies are the markers of dengue infection when antibody titres rise and virus is neutralized. Antibody based tests may also be suitable for seroprevalence and epidemiological surveillance. The combination of both antigen and antibody based tests in rapid kits and reference assay formats may counterbalance the advantages and disadvantages of standalone antigen or antibody based tests. Better differentiation between acute and convalescent phase of disease, primary and secondary dengue and epidemiological surveillance can be done. False positive results can be counterchecked as an inbuilt comparative control.

Combined Immunochromatography (Lateral Flow) (LF-ICT)

The LF-ICT contains dried antigens and colloidal gold-labelled monoclonal antibodies specific for dengue NS1, IgM and IgG on a nitrocellulose strip. IgA may also be included. A combined kit containing all of these increases the applicability in both acute and convalescent phase serum samples [78, 79, 80]. The high sensitivity, specificity and convenience of lateral flow immunochromatography in the present era have popularized its use in all healthcare settings. It is compact, faster to manufacture and has a prolonged shelf life. It can be carried out as a single bed-side test, in a single step, requires low sample volume and enables visual interpretation of results. The procedure eliminates use of electricity, washing step, contamination from reuse, sample pretreatment and laboratory infrastructure [81]. The applicability of either human, vector or environmental samples makes it universally employable as a frugal and robust diagnostic and epidemiological tool for both laboratory and field conditions, seroprevalence studies, mass screening programs and surveillance of dengue infections. There is no difference in detection with respect to different dengue serotypes, different viral loads or different clinical presentation.

The LF-ICT tests have been evaluated at airports to screen for imported dengue cases and also in peripheral/rural areas. Utilising Bayesian latent class models, wherein no test is assumed perfect, the sensitivity, specificity, PPV and NPV of combination NS1, IgM and IgG based tests have matched gold standards. It has been reported to differentiate 71% primary and 83% secondary dengue infections [80].

However, the results obtained are qualitative or semiquantitative, sensitivity is more for primary than secondary dengue, serotypes cannot be identified, and a negative result doesn't rule out dengue infection [82]. Further, there may be issues in generating a sensitive antibody with good selectivity and covalent attachment may decrease the affinity for the antigen [80]. The results of ELISA correlate well with that of LF-ICT, although the potential of a false positive IgM or IgG antibody due to the persistence of antibodies from a recent previous infection with a different dengue serotype or a related flavivirus should always be considered in endemic areas. [80]

REFERENCES

1. Chaturvedi UC, Agarwal R, Elbishbishi EA, Mustafa AS. Cytokine Cascade in Dengue Haemorrhagic Fever: Implications for Pathogenesis. *FEMS Immunol Med Microbiol.* 2000; 28:183-188.
2. Berry N, Chakravarti A, Gur R, Mathur MD. Serological investigation of a febrile outbreak in Delhi, India, using a rapid immunochromatographic test. J ClinMicrobiol. 1998; 36: 2795-2796.
3. Tripathi BK, Gupta B, Sinha RS, Prasad S, Sharma DK: Experience in adult population in dengue outbreak in Delhi. J Assoc Physicians India. 1998, 46:273-276.
4. Kumar M, Pasha ST, Mittal V, Rawat DS, Arya C, Agarwal N, et al. Unusual emergence of guate 98 like molecular subtype of Den -3 during 2003 dengue outbreak in Delhi. Dengue Bull. 2004; 28: 101-167.
5. Gubler DJ. Dengue and dengue hemorrhagic fever. ClinMicrobiol Rev. 1998; 11:480–496.
6. WHO: Strengthening implementation of the global strategy for dengue fever/dengue hemorrhagic fever prevention and control. Report on the informal consolation. WHO; 1999.
7. Vijayakumar TS, Chandy S, Sathish N, Abraham M, Abraham P, Sridharan G. Is dengue emerging as a major public health problem? Ind J Med Res. 2005; 121:100-107.
8. Vaughn DW, Kalayanarooj S, Innis BL, Nimmannitya S, et al. Dengue viremia titer, antibody response pattern, and virus serotype correlate with disease severity. J Infect Dis. 2000, 181:2-9.
9. Shu PY, et al. Development of group and serotype specific one-step SYBR Green I based real-time reverse transcription PCR assay for dengue virus. J ClinMicrobiol. 2003; 41: 2408–2416.
10. Halstead SB. Dengue hemorrhagic fever. A public health problem. WHO 1980; 58:1-21.
11. Malavige GN, Fernando DJ. Dengue infections. Postgrad Med J. 2004; 80: 588-601.
12. Harris E, Videa E, Perez L, Sandoval E, Tellez Y, Perez ML, et al. Clinical, epidemiologic, and virologic features of dengue in the 1998 epidemic in Nicaragua. Am J Trop Med Hyg. 2000; 63:5–11.

13. Pinheiro FP, Corber SJ: Global situation of dengue and dengue hemorrhagic fever, and its emergence in the Americas. World Health Stat Q. 1997, 50:161-169.
14. Libraty DH, Endy TP, Houng HS, Green S, Kalayanarooj S, et al. Differing influences of virus burden and immune activation on disease severity in secondary dengue-3 virus infections. J Infect Dis. 2002; 185: 1213–1221.
15. Messer WB, Gubler DJ, Harris E, Sivananthan K, de Silva AM: Emergence and global spread of a dengue serotype 3, subtype III virus. Emerg Infect Dis. 2003, 9:800-809.
16. Guzman MG, Kouri G. Dengue: An update. Lancet Infect Dis. 2002; 2:33-42.
17. WHO. Dengue hemorrhagic fever: diagnosis, treatment, prevention and control, 2nd edition. Geneva: World Health Organization 1997.
18. Broor S, Dar L, Sengupta S, Chakaraborty M, Wali JP, Biswas A, et al: Recent dengue epidemic in Delhi, India. In: Factors in the emergence of arbovirus diseases: Elsevier; 1997:P123-127.
19. Guzman MG, Kouri G, Bravo J, Valdes L, Vazquez S, Halstead SB: Effect of age on outcome of secondary dengue 2 infections. Int J Infect Dis. 2002, 6:118-124.
20. Chouhan GS, Rodrigues FM, Shaikh BH, Ilkal MA, Khangaro SS, Mathur KN, et al. Clinical & virological study of dengue fever outbreak in Jalore city, Rajasthan 1985. Ind J Med Res. 1990;91:414–418.
21. Padbidri VS, Mahadev PV, Thakre JP, Pant U, Illkal MA, Varghese GG, et al. Virological and entomological investigations of an outbreak of dengue fever in Dhule district, Maharashtra. Indian J Med Microbiol. 1996;14 : 25-32.
22. Mahadev PV, Kollali VV, Rawal ML, Pujara PK, Pathak V, Dhanda V, et al: Dengue in Gujarat state, India during 1988- 1989. Indian J Med Res. 1993, 97:135-144.
23. Bhattacharjee N, Mukherjee KK, Chakravarti SK, Mukherjee MK, De PN, Sengupta M, et al. Dengue hemorrhagic fever(DHF) outbreak in Calcutta-1990. J Commun Dis. 1993; 25: 10-4.
24. Idrees S, Ashfaq UA. A brief review on dengue molecular virology, diagnosis, treatment and prevalence in Pakistan. Genetic Vaccines and Therapy. 2012; 10 (6): 1-10.
25. Monath TP. Dengue: The risk to developed and developing countries. ProctlNatlAcadSci USA. 1994; 91:2395-2400.

26. Young PR, Hilditch PA, Bletchly C, Halloran W. An antigen capture enzyme-linked immunosorbent assay reveals high levels of the dengue virus protein NS1 in the sera of infected patients. J ClinMicrobiol. 2000;38:1053–1057.
27. Corwin AL, Larasati RP, Bangs MJ, WuryadiS,et al. Epidemic dengue transmission in southern Sumatra, Indonesia. Trans R Soc Trop Med Hyg. 2001, 95:257-265.
28. Bethell DB, Gamble J, Loc PP, Dung NM, Chau TTH, Loan HT, et al. Non-invasive measurement of microvascular leakage in patients with dengue hemorrhagic fever. Clin Infect Dis. 2001; 32: 243-253.
29. Sharma SN, Raina VK. Dengue: emerging disease in India. J Commun Dis. 2000; 32: 175-179.
30. Rosen L, Gubler D. The use of mosquitoes to detect and propagate dengue viruses. Am J Trop Med Hyg. 1974; 23:1153–1160.
31. Ko YC, Chen MJ, Yeh SM: The predisposing and protective factors against dengue virus transmission by mosquito vector. Am J Epidemiol. 1992; 136:214-220.
32. Muto RSA: Dengue Fever/DHF and its control - status in WHO's Western Pacific region by 1999. WHO report Manilla, WHO Western Pacific Regional Office; 2000:4.
33. Eram S, Setyabudi Y, Sadono TI, Gubler DJ, SuliantiSaroso J:Epidemic dengue hemorrhagic fever in rural Indonesia II. Clinical studies. Am J Trop Med Hyg. 1979, 28:711-716.
34. Mahadev PV, Kollali VV, Rawal ML, PujaraPK,et al. : Dengue in Gujarat state, India during 1988 & 1989. Indian J Med Res. 1993, 97:135-144.
35. Strickman D, Sithiprasasna R, Kittayapong P, Innis BL: Distribution of dengue and Japanese encephalitis among children in Thai villages. Am J Trop Med Hyg. 2000, 63:27-35.
36. Githeko AK, Lindsay SW, Confalonieri UE, Patz JA: Climate change and vector-borne diseases: a regional analysis. Bull World Health Organ. 2000; 78:1136-1147.
37. Shu PY, Huang JH. Current Advances in Dengue Diagnosis. Clin Vaccine Immunol. 2004; 11 (4):642-650.
38. Guzman MG, Halstead SB, Artsob H, Buchy P, Farrar J, Gubler DJ, et al. Dengue: a continuing global threat. Nat Rev Microbiol. 2010;8:S7–16.
39. Martina BE, Koraka P, Osterhaus AD. Dengue virus pathogenesis: an integrated view. ClinMicrobiol Rev. 2009; 22 (4): 564–581.

40. Agarwal R, Kapoor S, Nagar R, Misra A, Tandon R, Mathur A, et al: A clinical study of the patients with dengue hemorrhagic fever of 1996 at Lucknow, India. Southeast Asian J Trop Med Public Health. 1999; 30:735-740.
41. Goh KT, Ng SK, Chan YC, Lim SJ, Chua EC: Epidemiological aspects of an outbreak of DF/DHF in Singapore. Southeast Asian J Trop Med Public Health. 1987; 18:295-302.
42. Halstead SB, Nimmannitya S, Cohen SN: Observations related to pathogenesis of dengue hemorrhagic fever. IV. Relation of disease severity to antibody response and virus recovered. Yale J Biol Med. 1970; 42:311-328
43. Whitehorn J, Farrar J. Dengue. Br Med Bull. 2010; 95:161-173.
44. Sa-Ngasand A, Anantapreecha S, A-Nuegoonpipat A, Chanama S, Wibulwattanakij S, Pattanakul K, et al. Specific IgM and IgG responses in primary and secondary dengue virus infections determined by enzyme-linked immunosorbent assay. Epidemiology and Infection. 2006; 134(4):820–825.
45. Gubler DJ, Sather GE. Laboratory diagnosis of dengue and dengue hemorrhagic fever. In: Homma A, Cunha JF, editors. Proceedings of the International Symposium on Yellow Fever and Dengue. 1988; 291–322.
46. Koraka P, Suharti C, Setiati TE, Mairuhu ATA, Gorp EV, Hack CE etal. Kinetics of Dengue Virus-Specific Serum Immunoglobulin Classes and Subclasses Correlate with Clinical Outcome of Infection. J ClinMicrobiol. 2001; 39(12):4332-4338.
47. Halstead SB, Nimmannitya S, Cohen SN: Observations related to pathogenesis of dengue hemorrhagic fever. Yale J Biol Med. 1970; 42:311-328.
48. Halstead SB. DHF: A public health problem. Bull WHO. 1980; 58:1-21.
49. Ooi EE, Hart TJ, Tan HC: Dengue seroepidemiology in Singapore. Lancet. 2001, 357:685-686.
50. Halstead SB, Rourke EJ. Dengue viruses and mononuclear phagocytes. Infection enhancement by non-neutralizing antibody. J Exp Med. 1977; 146: 201-217.
51. Morens DM, Rigau-Perez JG, Lopez-Correa RH, et al.: Dengue in Puerto Rico, 1977: public health response to characterize and control an epidemic of multiple serotypes. Am J Trop Med Hyg. 1986; 35:197-211.

52. Guzman MG, Kouri GP, Bravo J, Soler M, Vazquez S, Morier L: Dengue hemorrhagic fever in Cuba, 1981: a retrospective seroepidemiologic study. Am J Trop Med Hyg. 1990, 42:179-184.
53. Churdboonchart V, Bhamarapravati N, Peampramprecha S, Sirinavin S. Antibodies against dengue viral proteins in primary and secondary dengue hemorrhagic fever. Am J Trop Med Hyg. 1991; 44:481–493.
54. Bhamarapravati N, Toochinda P, Boonyapaknavik V. Pathology of Thailand hemorrhagic fever: a study of 100 autopsy cases. Ann Trop Med Parasitol. 1967; 61(4): 500-510.
55. Narayanan M, Aravind MA, Thilothammal N, Prema R, Sargunam CS, Ramamurty N, et al. Dengue fever epidemic in Chennai – A study of clinical profile and outcome. Indian Pediatr. 2002; 39: 1027-33.
56. Kamath SR, Ranjit S. Clinical features, complications and atypical manifestations of children with severe forms of DHF in South India. Indian J Pediatr. 2006; 73(10):889-895.
57. Rasul CH, Ahasan HA, Rasid AK, Khan MR: Epidemiological factors of dengue hemorrhagic Fever in Bangladesh. Indian Pediatr. 2002; 39: 369-372.
58. Kuno G, Gomez I, Gubler D J. An ELISA procedure for the diagnosis of dengue infections. J Virol Methods. 1991; 33:101–113.
59. Peeling RW, Artsob H, Pelegrino JL, Buchy P, Cardosa MJ, Devi S, et al. Evaluation of diagnostic tests: dengue. Nature Reviews Microbiology. 2013; S30-S37.
60. Vaughn DW, Green S, Kalayanarooj S, Innis BL, Nimmannitya S, Suntayakorn S, et al. Dengue in the early febrile phase: viremia and antibody responses. J Infect Dis. 1997; 176:322–330.
61. Sahni AK, Grover N, Sharma A, Khan ID, Kishore J. Reverse transcription loop-mediated isothermal amplification (RT-LAMP) for diagnosis of dengue. Medical Journal Armed Forces India (2012), http://dx.doi.org/10.1016/j.mjafi.2012.07.017. [E- pub ahead of print].
62. Kuno G. Universal diagnostic RT-PCR protocol for arboviruses. J Virol Methods. 1998; 72:27–41.
63. Lanciotti RS, Calisher CH, Gubler DJ, Chang GJ, Vorndam AV. Rapid detection and typing of dengue viruses from clinical samples by using reverse transcriptase-polymerase chain reaction. J ClinMicrobiol. 1992; 30:545–551.

64. Leone G, van Schijndel H, van Gemen B, Kramer FR, Schoen CD. Molecular beacon probes combined with amplification by NASBA enable homogeneous, real-time detection of RNA. Nucleic Acids Res. 1998; 26: 2150–2155.
65. Seah CLL, Chow VTK, Tan HC, Chan YC. Rapid single-step RT-PCR typing of dengue viruses using NS3 gene primers. J Virol Methods. 1995; 51:193–200.
66. Sudiro TM, Ishiko H, Green S, Vaughn DW, Nisalak A, Kalayanarooj S, et al. Rapid diagnosis of dengue viremia by reverse transcriptasepolymerase chain reaction using 3_-noncoding region universal primers. Am J Trop Med Hyg.1997; 56:424–429.
67. Henchal EA, McCown JM, Seguin MC, Gentry MK, Brandt WE. Rapid identification of dengue virus isolates by using monoclonal antibodies in an indirect immunofluorescence assay. Am J Trop Med Hyg. 1983; 32:164–169.
68. Da Fonseca BA, Fonseca SN: Dengue virus infections. CurrOpinPediatr. 2002, 14:67-71.
69. Mackay IM, Arden KE, Nitsche A. Real-time PCR in virology. Nucleic Acids Res.2002; 30: 1292 –1305.
70. Wang WK, Sung TL, Tsai YC, Chang SM, King CC. Detection of dengue virus replication in peripheral blood mononuclear cells from dengue virus type 2-infected patients by a reverse transcription-real-time PCR assay. J ClinMicrobiol. 2002; 40:4472–4478.
71. Harris ET, Roberts G, Smith L, Selle J, Kramer LD, Valle S, et al. Typing of dengue viruses in clinical specimens and mosquitoes by single-tube multiplex reverse transcriptase PCR. J ClinMicrobiol. 1998; 36:2634–2639.
72. Berry N, Chakravarti A, Gur R, Mathur MD. Serological investigation of a febrile outbreak in Delhi, India, using a rapid immunochromatographic test. J ClinMicrobiol. 1998; 36: 2795-2796.
73. Notomi T, Okayama H, Masubuchi H, Yonekawa T, Watanabe K, Amino N, et al. Loop-mediated isothermal amplification of DNA. Nucleic Acids Research. 2000;28:E63–e63.
74. Samuel PP, Tyagi BK. Diagnostic methods for detection and isolation of dengue viruses from vector mosquitoes. Indian J Med Res. 2006; 123: 615-628.
75. Guzman MG, Kouri G. Advances in dengue diagnosis. ClinDiagn Lab Immunol. 1996; 3: 621–627.

76. Callahan JD, Wu SJ, Dion-Schultz A, Mangold BE, Peruski LF, Watts DM, et al. Development and evaluation of serotype and group-specific fluorogenic reverse transcriptase PCR (TaqMan) assays for dengue virus. J ClinMicrobiol. 2001; 39:4119–4124.
77. Houng HH, Chen RCM, Vaughn DW, Kanesa-thasan N. Development of a fluorogenic RT-PCR system for quantitative identification of dengue virus serotypes 1–4 using conserved and serotype-specific 3_noncoding sequences. J Virol Methods. 2001; 95:19–32.
78. Osorio L, Ramirez M, Bonelo A, Villar LA, Parra B. Comparison of the diagnostic accuracy of commercial NS1-based diagnostic tests for early dengue infection. Virology Journal. 2010, 7:361.
79. Blacksell SD, Jarman RG, Bailey MS, Tanganuchitcharnchai A, Janjaroen K, Gibbons RV, et al. Evaluation of Six Commercial Point-of-Care Tests for Diagnosis of Acute Dengue Infections: the Need for Combining NS1 Antigen and IgM/IgG Antibody Detection To Achieve Acceptable Levels of Accuracy. Clin Vaccine Immunol. 2011; 18(12): 2095–2101.
80. Khan ID, Sahni AK. Rapid Diagnosis of Dengue Outbreaks in Resource Limited Facilities. West Indian Medical Journal. 2016. E-pub ahead of print. 10:7727/wimj.2016.095
81. Posthuma-Trumpie GA, Korf J. The high sensitivity, specificity and convenience of lateral flow immunochromatography in the present era have popularized its use in all healthcare settings. Anal Bioanal Chem. 2009; 393:569–582.
82. Hang VT, Nguyet NM, Trung DT, Tricou V, Yoksan S, Dung NM, et al. Diagnostic accuracy of NS1 ELISA and lateral flow rapid tests for dengue sensitivity, specificity and relationship to viraemia and antibody responses. PLoSNegl Trop Dis. 2009;3:e360.